PSYCHIATRIES' PRESUMPTIONS:
A Portuguese Historic-cultural Perspective

PSYCHIATRIES' PRESUMPTIONS:
A Portuguese Historic-cultural Perspective

By

J.A. Zagallo-Cardoso
M.D., M. Med. Sc., Ph. D. (University of Coimbra, Portugal)

Strategic Book Publishing and Rights Co.

© 2015 by J.A. Zagallo-Cardoso, M.D., M. Med. Sc., Ph. D.
All rights reserved.

No part of this book may be reproduced or transmitted in any form or by any means, graphic, electronic, or mechanical, including photocopying, recording, taping, or by any information storage retrieval system, without the permission, in writing, from the publisher. For more information, send a letter to our Houston, TX address, Attention Subsidiary Rights Department, or email: mailto:support@sbpra.net.

Strategic Book Publishing and Rights Co.
12620 FM 1960, Suite A4-507
Houston, TX 77065
www.sbpra.com

For information about special discounts for bulk purchases, please contact Strategic Book Publishing and Rights Co. Special Sales, at bookorder@sbpra.net

ISBN: 978-1-63135-697-1

Book Design by Julius Kiskis

22 21 22 20 19 18 17 16 15   1 2 3 4 5

Dedication

Dedicated to Professor Alexander Frederic Jenner,
with fond respect to our inspiriting master.

Contents

Preface ix

Acknowledgments xi

1. The Natural-Scientific, Anthropophilosophical, And Transcultural Implications Of The Portuguese Discoveries 1

2. Discoveries Of Some Portuguese Personalities Relevant To Psychiatric Thought 4

3. Fernando Pessoa (1888–1935), The Portuguese "Philosopher-Poet" And Psychiatrist 12

4. Psychiatrizing Society And Panopticism 25

Glossary 39

Bibliography 41

Preface

This work endorses four ideas that can be globally considered one autonomous point of view about psychiatry; that is, a view that tries to dismiss a presumption of psychiatry. My paper analyzes these ideas, reviews them critically, and concludes with a perspective on "panopticism."

The European philosopher who, for better or worse, had the most influence on the directions of contemporary psychiatry is unanimously acknowledged to be Karl Jaspers. The following are direct quotes from Jaspers:

"Philosophy doesn't have, as science does, a characteristic of progressive process."

"We are definitely ahead of Hippocrates, the Greek doctor. However, we cannot say that we are ahead of Plato, except in regard to the amount of scientific knowledge and material that he had at hand. Philosophically speaking, we probably haven't reached his level."

Despite the implications of evolutionist epistemology, this method of situating philosophy has nothing to do with parallelism between natural and cultural evolutions. It brings to mind the necessary scientific humility by recognizing that the older interrogations of Man concerning himself continue to be great interrogations of modern Man.

There is a "political conflict" about what is sacred and what is mad, especially when faced with borderline life, artistic creation, and love. The social collective is forced to define itself in the light of discordances. It must confront them in the fundamentals of its own culture. It responds by domesticating.

The main parts of this work are the following:

I. The natural-scientific, anthropophilosophical, and transcultural implications of the Portuguese discoveries.

II. Discoveries of some Portuguese personalities relevant to psychiatric thought.

III. Fernando Pessoa (1888–1935), the Portuguese "philosopher-poet" and psychiatrist.

IV. Psychiatrizing society and panopticism

Acknowledgments

We are grateful to Professor Alec Jenner for his enthusiastic help and involvement in this work, which has been yet another happy Anglo-Portuguese venture. We also thank the British Council (Lisbon) and the Fundação Oriente (Lisbon) for their help and support.

1.
The Natural-Scientific, Anthropophilosophical, and Transcultural Implications of the Portuguese Discoveries

The Portuguese sea discoveries (fifteenth and sixteenth centuries) made possible a wide range of data relative to fauna and flora; to meteorological phenomena, such as aerial and naval currents, the tides and their courses, climate, and geography; the races of people, their habitat, their religion and traditions, their commerce, their civil and military organization, etc. All this constructed other stimuli for the development of observation, which until then had been suffocated, in part by the custom of regarding all phenomenal wonders of nature as prodigies. It is this progressively enriched habit of observation that permitted us to learn essential concepts.

The route to those concepts presents some well-defined characteristics that Professor Luis de Albuquerque referred to in the following way:

1. Firstly, when we study the nautical texts of that time, we immediately see that "men connected to maritime life not only expressly recognized the practical value of observation, but also managed to think a few times of reproducing phenomena

artificially, or 'through art' (in the Aristotelian sense of expression), as a way to better the studies or to justify what was supposedly established about them..."

2. Secondly, "the experience demanded skill in the systematic observations, so the sailors perfected their qualities as observers in the most difficult way possible with such primitive methods..."

3. Thirdly, "in the beginning the observation ended up underlining the value of the analogy as a way to progress in the objective knowledge of the world, and the cinquecentist sailor didn't stop using it in that manner even though there were true consequences from it..."

4. Fourthly, "the observations registered during those trips demanded the profound development of the critical spirit that until then had been ignored. However, these observations weren't generally considered secondary aspects or marginal problems..."

5. Lastly, "the navigators also learnt to doubt certain teachings transmitted by the classics, an attitude that stood out when all of Europe was certainly dominated by a current of valorization of the scientific knowledge of antiquity. This is what Duarte Pacheco Pereira did in the Esmeraldo, improving what had been written about Africa by Ptolomeu, Pomponio Mela, Plinio, and other geographers..."

> Therefore, "in a polarized intellectual climate, these fundamental ideas were necessary to open access lines into a type of positive thought: and this is what really happened, but not as easily as we first thought. In reality, man is somewhat a prisoner of the mental outlines in which he lives, and only through a drawn-out fight can he liberate himself from the preconceptions that have evolved around him. In the threshold of the sixteenth century, the

Portuguese-European men reached a crossroad: it was proposed that they switch a world somewhat in order, that they lived in with its laws, and that had only begun to show its most evident deficiencies for another world that wasn't yet perfectly defined, that in a certain way looked chaotic, and that was reasonably supposed to be full of surprises. In all the decisive steps of the history of human thought the situation has been the same, and man, because of his love for adventure, has always won in his choice of the apparently disturbed road that will conduct him to the most ample perspectives."

The European imagination changed with the Portuguese discoveries. Initial information about Brazil and its native people—wrongly called Indians by the Spanish because C. Colombo thought that he had arrived in India and he forbade his crew to say anything contrary to this idea, threatening to cut their tongues—lead to the building of social ideals and myths in translated works such as those of Thomas More (Utopia) and Jean Jaques Rousseau (The Good Savage).

In the abstract, we could synthesize all those aspects in the sense of Luís Vaz de Camões: "knowledge made from the experience . . ." (in Portuguese: "O saber de experiência feito . . ."). And, consequently, we can say with Fernando Pessoa that "the most relevant discovery of the Portuguese was the discovery of the idea of discovery."

2.
DISCOVERIES OF SOME PORTUGUESE PERSONALITIES RELEVANT TO PSYCHIATRIC THOUGHT

The Islamic presence in Portugal (eighth through thirteenth centuries) lasted longer than the Roman domination and was very rich in psychological knowledge, with well-known names such as Avicena (Ibn Siña) or Averroes, classic doctors of the peninsular culture.

We should mention two authors from the Middle Ages: São Martinho de Dume and Pedro Hispano.

From Bracara (Braga) religious and philosophical tradition, we mention São Martinho de Dume (518?–79), Bishop of Braga and then of Dume, his own cathedral, who was inspired by Séneca and wrote about passions, virtues, sins, and how to deal with them. He wrote Da Ira (On Anger): its nature, its causes, its effects and its management. He wrote, "Do not let yourself be carried away by the authority of the speaker. Concentrate not on who is speaking but on what he says." He preceded psychophysics by studying "anatomically" the passions and the influence of attitudes on behavior.

The notable contribution of Pedro Hispano (Petrus Hispanus, 1200–1277), a doctor and philosopher originally from Lisbon, is mentioned in Dante's Divine Comedy (1304–1324). Hispanus, who became Pope John XXI in 1276, viewed psychology as the pars nobilissima of nature and maintained that the study of such phenomena belonged to the natural sciences rather than to philosophy. Hispanus foresaw, with remarkable accuracy, modern views of "psychosomatic medicine." His fundamental text of philosophical psychology, "Comments," on Aristotle's De Anima, was found in Madrid (eighteenth century).

From the Renaissance we distinguish a pioneer in the hospital treatment of mental patients, João Cidade (1495–1550), who later became Saint John of God. He was born in Montemor-oVelho, near Évora, and worked mainly in Andaluzia, near Valencia. He founded the first Asylum in the world (at Valencia) and created the Religious Order of Hospitallers. Since then, this order has contributed to the creation of many other asylums (future psychiatric hospitals) throughout the world. The charitable treatment – gentle and occupational – introduced by São João de Deus constituted a real revolution in relation to the cruel manner in which insane people had been treated until then.

The Portuguese king, Dom Duarte I (1391–1438), "The Eloquent King," through deep introspection and an autobiographical approach, wrote the world's first exhaustive description of melancholia (depression). He described its beginning, characteristics (symptoms), development, and cure by auto-treatment in his book Leal Conselheiro (1438), a treatise on ethics and morals to be read by court members.

Among the scientists of the discoveries period, we mention Dr. Garcia d'Orta (1501/2–1568), pioneer of tropical medicine, in the opinion of the historian Charles Boxer. Garcia d'Orta wrote an emblematic book for modern pharmacology, Colóquiodos dos Simples e Drogas da Índia, which describes many psychological effects of the plants that he studied.

Some Portuguese medical doctors dedicated relevant attention to psychological phenomena in their works. These doctors included Amatus Lusitanos (João Rodrigues Castelo Branco) (1511–68); Francisco Sanches (1551–1623); and António Nunes Ribeiro Sanches (1699-1783), who was physician to the Russian czarina Ana Ivanovna. The pedagogue Luís António Vernay (1713–1792) wrote on the passions of the soul.

We can say that "psychoanalysis as therapeutic method did not originate with Sigmund Freud" (Cardoso, 1952). Amongst the precursors of Freud, through the practice of "Lucide Sleep," an intermediate concept between the "animal magnetism" of Mesmer and the future "therapeutic hypnosis" of James Braid (1795–1860), we have the Portuguese doctor Abade de Faria (1756–1819), licensed in Portuguese India (Estado da Índia), who would later emigrate from Lisbon to Paris. This somewhat legendary personality was praised by Alexander Dumas as one of the main characters of his romance The Count of Monte Cristo. Abade de Faria criticized Mesmer's myth of "animal magnetism" and interpreted it as a psychological phenomenon. This explanation became noteworthy when it emerged in the era of mechanistic materialism. One of Faria's students, in Paris was J. M. Charcot (1825–93), of Iberian descent, with whom Sigmund Freud (1856–1939) learned hypnosis a few years later.

As a consequence of the Inquisition many Portuguese Jews emigrated to other countries. Among them were some relevant personalities of the humanities and even of medicine and philosophy. We will refer to two of these men.

Bento Baruch de Espinoza (1632–77) originated from a Portuguese Judaic family from Algarve that took refuge in Holland. The work of this "thinker" must not be ignored in the humanistic formation of psychological and psychiatric professionals. Espinoza described the psychophysics unity of men. Espinoza's system is a rationalistic model with a base in the mystical experience of unity in the multiplicity and under the sign of eternity. Espinoza's psychology is of the eternal present. He admits that the force of passions disappears in the presence of reason, but he considers the power of reason transitory. The spiritual revolution that he proposes is a bet on any mechanistic model. Espinoza aspired to construct a society that permitted the majority of people to acquire a supreme light.

The North American Jacob Mendes da Costa (1883–1900) also originated from Portugal and belonged to a Judaic family. His description (1871) of the irritable heart syndrome is certainly a notable achievement percussive on the modern concept of the psychosomatic.

The attempt at surgical treatments of mental patients, suggestively designated psycho-surgery, brought up philosophical problems of great significance. In 1935 the Portuguese neurologist Egas Moniz (1874–1955), inspired by the work of Ramon y Cajal and the physiology of Pavlov, attributed the organic basis of thought to the synapses. He tried to deduce from the therapeutic effects of prefrontal leucotomy, for which discovery he won the Nobel Prize in 1949, that certain psychoses, including schizophrenia, were caused by abnormal brain function. Szasz (1977) commented on this inference that Moniz recognized that his objective in applying leucotomy to human beings was less to find a cure for psychoses than to lay the cornerstone for the edifice of organic psychiatry. That meant to establish a firm basis for an organic theory of the functional psychoses. I cite the work of Egas Moniz not to condemn him but to illustrate why this type of investigation is unlike traditional medical research. In order to establish the organic nature of dementia paralytica, the medical research workers studied postmortem brains. Hence they established the histopathological nature of the condition. They had not tried to prove that G.P.I. was an organic disease mutilating the body nor to draw conclusions from the therapeutic intervention about the nature of the disease. The reasoning behind the method of Egas Moniz is widely accepted today. For instance, it is generally believed that because the fact that the major tranquilizers affect behavior in desirable ways proves that patients have a disease with an organic base. Of course Moniz, a neurologist, did not conduct a unique surgical intervention. On the other hand, he had an arthrosis that prevented him from doing so. They were made by the Portuguese neurosurgeon Almeida Lima. It is important to remember that leucotomy has nothing to do with the aggressive lobotomy practiced in the United States by Freeman et al. When discussing Egas Moniz, it would not be fair to omit his discovery of cerebral angiography, which had an unquestionable clinical interest until the development of neuroimaging techniques.

António Rosa Damásio was born in Lisbon on February 25, 1944. He studied medicine at the University of Lisbon Medical School, where he also completed his neurological residency and his doctorate. He worked as a research fellow at the Aphasia Research Center in Boston in 1967, prior to receiving his MD in Lisbon. He worked there on behavioral neurology, under the supervision of the late Norman Geschwind, the Harvard neurologist who created the field.

As a researcher, Damásio was most interested in the neurobiology of the mind. He was especially interested in neural systems that subserve memory, language, emotion, decision-making, and consciousness. He showed that emotions and their biological underpinnings are involved in decision-making (both positively and negatively, and often unconsciously); provide the scaffolding for the construction of social cognition; and are required for the self-processes which undergird consciousness.

It is often discussed in peer-review experimental and theoretical work (an index of its relevance can be gleaned from the fact that the Institute of Scientific Information has named Damásio as one of the most highly cited researchers in the past decade). Damásio has formulated the somatic markers hypothesis, which captures the essence of these ideas. Current work on the biology of moral decisions, neuro-economics, social communication, and drug-addiction, has been strongly influenced by Damásio's hypothesis.

Damásio also proposed that emotions are part of homeostatic regulation and are rooted in reward/punishment mechanisms. He recovered James's perspective on feelings as a read-out of body states but expanded it with an "as-if-body-loop" device that allows the substrate of feelings to be simulated rather than actual (foreshadowing the simulation process later uncovered by mirror neurons). He demonstrated experimentally that the insular cortex is a critical platform for feelings, a finding that has been widely replicated, and he uncovered cortical and subcortical induction sites for human emotions, e.g., in ventromedial prefrontal cortex and amygdala.

In another development, Damásio proposed that the cortical architecture on which learning and recall depend involves multiple, hierarchically organized loops of axonal projections that converge on certain nodes out of which projections diverge to the points of origin of convergence (the convergence-divergence framework). This architecture is applicable to the understanding of memory processes and of aspects of consciousness related to the access of mental contents.

In "The Feeling of What Happens," Damásio lays the foundations of the "enchainment of precedences," namely, "the unconscious neural signaling of an individual organism begets the protoself which permits core self and core consciousness, which allow for an autobiographical self, which permits extended consciousness. At the end of the chain, extended consciousness permits conscience."

Damásio's research depended significantly on establishing the modern human lesion method, an enterprise made possible by Hanna Damásio's structural neuroimaging/neuroanatomy work complemented by experimental neuroanatomy (with Gary Van Hoesen and Josef Parvizi), experimental neuropsychology (with Antoine Bechara, Ralph Adolphs, and Dan Tranel), and functional neuroimaging (with Kaspar Meyer, Jonas Kaplan, and Mary Helen Immordino-Yang).

As clinicians, he and his collaborators have studied and treated disorders of behavior and cognition, and movement disorders.

Damásio's books deal with the relationship between emotions and feelings and what their bases may be within the brain. His 1994 book, *Descartes' Error*: Emotion, Reason and the Human Brain, won the Science et Vie prize, was a finalist for the Los Angeles Times Book Award, and has been translated into over thirty languages. It is regarded as one of the most influential books of the past two decades. His second book, The Feeling of What Happens: Body and Emotion in the Making of Consciousness, was named as one of the ten best books of 2001 by the New York Times Book Review, was a Publishers Weekly Best Book of the Year, was a Library Journal Best Book of the Year, and has over thirty foreign editions. Damásio's Looking for Spinoza: Joy, Sorrow, and the Feeling Brain was published in 2003. In it, Damásio suggested that the protobiologist Spinoza's thinking foreshadowed discoveries in biology and neuroscience views on the mind-body problem. His latest book is Self Comes to Mind: Constructing the Conscious Brain. In it Damásio suggests that the self is the key to conscious minds and that feelings, from the kind he designates as primordial to the well-known feelings of emotion, are the basic elements in the construction of the protoself and core self.

Damásio is a member of the American Academy of Arts and Sciences, the National Academy of Sciences' Institute of Medicine, and the European Academy of Sciences and Arts. Damásio has received many awards, including the Prince of Asturias Award in Science and Technology, the Kappers Neuroscience Medal, the Beaumont Medal from the American Medical Association, the Nonino Prize, the Reenpaa Prize in Neuroscience, and, most recently, the Honda Prize. He has received honorary doctoral degrees (Doctor honoris causa) from the University of Aachen (2002), University of Aveiro (2003), University of Copenhagen (Copenhagen Business School, 2009), University of Leiden (2010), University Ramon Llull, Barcelona (2010), University of Coimbra (2011), and the Swiss Federal Institute of Technology, Lausanne (2011).

His current work involves the social emotions, consciousness, and the creative interface between neuroscience and the arts, especially music and film. Despite or because of that fallibilism, Damásio writes in the belief that "scientific knowledge can be a pillar to help humans endure and prevail."

3.
Fernando Pessoa (1888-1935) The Portuguese "Philosopher-Poet" and Psychiatrist

The unanimously acknowledged European philosopher who had the greatest influence, for better or worse, on contemporary psychiatry was Karl Jaspers (1883–1969). He wrote:

"Philosophy doesn't have, as science does, a progressive character . . . We are definitely ahead of Hippocrates, the Greek doctor. However, we cannot say that we are ahead of Plato, except in regard to the amount of scientific knowledge and material that he had at hand. Philosophically speaking, we probably haven't reached his level."

When Professor Alec Jenner, from Sheffield, asked us to discuss Pessoa and psychiatry, we were brought face to face, despite the truth of Jaspers's comments, with the need for scientific humility in regard to the art of living. Modern poetry may not have outstripped Homer, not music Mozart, but neither they nor philosophy can therefore be dismissed. It is valuable to be reminded of the relevance of the ancient's enquiries into man's being, but clearly they must be remembered in ways that help modern people with their own enquiries. Hence we thank

Professor Jenner for his initiative in setting up this discussion. In a book we have written jointly with him, we discuss critically and in some detail Jaspers's impact on psychiatry (Schizophrenia A disease or Some Ways of Being Human? Sheffield Academic Press). As the later Wittgenstein would have it, and as we suspect Jaspers would too, language does not just describe the world. It has many other functions, such as commanding, pleading, and creating social and human reality. There is also a question of what descriptive science is. Furthermore, our lives are inauthentic if we don't see how much of our thinking must be outside of even apparently objective description. Perhaps the complex genius of the poet, Pessoa, illustrates this and he would have enjoyed our paradoxical position of attempting to say what is so by asserting that there is often much wrong with believing one can do so!

Since we are from Portugal, we would like to outline another motive for you: the thought of a poet. Portugal has often been referred to as a land of poets. Portugal's National Day is not the day of a king, a politician, or a warrior, but the day of Luis de Camões, the poet who depicted the Portuguese Discoveries.

The etymology of the Greek work "Poiesis" takes us to the notion of doing. And the poet is precisely he "who does." The Iberian poetry of the Golden Century (sixteenth century) functioned as a cultural influence, and the poets were especially aware of the language. In that era, poetry, the art of doing, served three fundamental purposes: registering, functioning, and inventing the world.

Fernando Pessoa (1888–1935) is usually considered Portugal's greatest modern poet, with an international standing identical to that of Camões (Portugal's Shakespeare). The German poet Hölderlin (1770–1843), so admired and quoted by Heidegger (1889–1976), wrote that poets and philosophers live in mountains separated by a deep abyss. It seems, however, that it is not so rare to find poets who co-inhabit the mountain of the philosophers or at least join the two mountains with bridges that cross the ontological gap. Pessoa, one of the most original European poets in the twentieth century, deserves, without doubt, the epithet of "philosopher-poet." His intense preoccupation with the nature of human existence and with our relation to the universe was coupled with an austere and even cold but striking originality. He was a withdrawn, quiet, and enigmatic person, obviously providing discussion material for psychiatrists.

Pessoa's father died when he was five, and his stepfather was the Portuguese consul in Durban. Pessoa was educated in English in South Africa and wrote his early works and some of his later works in English. In 1903, at the age of fifteen, he received the Queen Victoria Award in English Composition at the University of Cape of Good Hope after his entrance examination. He was familiar with and much influenced by English literature (the works of Shakespeare, Byron, Milton, Poe, Keats, Tennyson, Wordsworth, etc.), and its American counterpart, especially works by Walt Whitman.

After school he returned to Portugal and started, but never completed, a University course. Whether he was content with it or not, he spent most of his life living on a low income, translating for a commercial firm. This didn't take much of his time, so he was able to devote himself to his obsessive study or being human.

There is often a sense of Schopenhauer's Terror of Existence in Pessoa's writings, but it is coupled with a great ability to write as many quite different people. Pessoa had more than sixty personas. He used his own name as well, but his four principal personas, or imaginary people, were: Alberto Caeiro, Ricardo Reis, Alvaro de Campos, and Bernando Soares. The first three of these personas were preoccupied with metaphysical difficulties, but each from a self-consistent yet different standpoint. Some of Pessoa's other pseudonyms were English poets, such as Alexander Search.

Pessoa made his own existence a live poem. He wrote of his persona creation: "It's a drama made of people, instead of acts." He incarnated the drama of human existence under the formula of those various contradictory personas, each a gifted, animated, and proper personality with his own biography. The personas polarized different facets and categories. This is the human universality and singularity, the irrational and rational, the absolute and relative, the revolt and nostalgia, the solitude and gregariousness, the paradoxes and ambiguity, the modern and traditional . . . .

His name, Pessoa (person in English), comes from the Greek word persona, which means mask. Pessoa clearly perceived us as multiple personalities and joyfully recommended, "Be plural as is the Universe!"

Bachlard wrote that "we don´t do poetry inside a unity; the unity has no poetic capacity."

Here was no concept of the unity of the ego and self, which is assumed by phenomenologists and in common sense. This, among other features, has made Pessoa a subject of psychiatric enquiries. However, here we are less interested in psychiatrists' attempts to understand art and artists than in the writer's legitimate and illuminating comments on psychiatry and psychopathology. Hence we are concerned with Pessoa's comments and reflections on psychiatry and his diagnoses of the human state. In a sense he made it clear that he saw psychopathology as a socially legitimated ideology that meant little ontologically:

> "In reality the unique critics of art and literature ought to be the psychiatrists; they are as ignorant and remote from these issues and from what they call

science as other people; nevertheless, when faced with mental disease, they have the competence that our judgment says they have. No body of human knowledge can be built on any other basis" (1915).

It is clear that Pessoa conceptualized mankind quite differently than Aristotle. As Pessoa wrote: ". . . Man is an irrational animal, exactly as all others . . . .Man doesn't know more than other animals; he knows less. They know what they need to know; we don't." Also, ". . . Emotion and not reason control Man as it does animals . . . science and reason presiding as a constitutional monarch, who reigns but doesn't govern. Human action is irrational, contradictory, and absurd . . . reason illuminates a way; it doesn't determine."

This implies that the decoding of most so-called symptoms probably goes beyond the limits of an official psychopathology and common sense. Man the plural being, who is self-contradictory and alienated from his own experiences, requires us to revise our conceptions of human being (perhaps Heidegger's Dasein) and the methods of the human sciences. "Only when this is done can the true meaningfulness of mad behavior become apparent . . . and at the same time the true madness of behavior which common sense takes to be sane" (Ingleby, 1981).

On Freud, Pessoa wrote:

"The European and ultra-European success of Freud proceeds, in my view, in part from the originality of the criteria, in part because this has the force and narrowness of madness (this is how religions and religious cults are formed, because they are the political mysticisms such as fascism, communism, and others such as these), but especially from the criteria based on a sexual interpretation (with some exceptions by some followers). This gives way to absolutely obscene books that have been written as titles of scientific works (that sometimes are), which can 'interpret' past and present artists and writers in a degrading sense; in a Brazilian form the 'Chiado' style. That way of administering psychic masturbation in the vast network of onanisms that seem to form the contemporary civilization's mentality (. . .) that was the detail that created the great interest in Freudianism all over the world and for that reason publicized the system."

And he continued:

"Freudianism is an imperfect system (. . .) if we think that it will give us the key that no other system can give us about the undefined complexity of the human soul" (1931).

Pessoa is always skeptical, informed, insightful, and mystical, and he is usually intentionally paradoxical. Life is vital and mysterious; the reduction to the mechanical or adequately explicable is the denial of artistry, which deals with paradoxical truths eternally beyond scientific reduction, however valuable the latter may be.

In his poem "Dom Sebastian, King of Portugal" (who suffered massive defeat at Alcazar-Kebir, in 1578, at the hands of the Moroccans), Pessoa encapsulates the dread of the reality he attempts to grasp and the fears that, in a Sartrean sense, nauseate him.

DOM SEBASTIAN, KING OF PORTUGAL

Mad; yes Mad, because I desired greatness
Such as fate does not give
I couldn't contain my certainty within me;
That's why, where the sandy shore is,
My being-that-was remained – not the one that is.

My madness, let others accept it from me,
And all that it contained
Without madness what is man
Other than a healthy animal,
An adjourned and procreating corpse?

In another poem he also seems to capture something approaching the passive feelings of the schizophrenic, or at least the human reality of being a product as much as an agent:

Sudden hand of some hidden ghost
Among the folds of night and of my sleep
Shakes me awake, and in the forsakenness of night
I glimpse neither gesture nor shape
But an ancient terror, unburied in my heart
Descends from its throne
To affirm itself my lord master:
Without order, without nod, without insult

And I feel my life all of a sudden
Caught by a rope of unawareness
In some nocturnal hand which guides me

I feel that I am no one but a shadow
Of a shape I cannot see which haunts me
And I exist in nothing like the cold dark

Keeping in mind how Pessoa perceived the myth (he writes that "myth is nothing that is all"), we return to a Portuguese preoccupation with King Sebastian. A Portuguese myth anticipated and desired the return of the king. Pessoa wrote that they should believe "whether or not he returns." Here he is highlighting the acceptability of strange and ridiculous (socially valued) views as opposed to socially rejected opinions (psychiatry's delusions). Beliefs, he is implying, have values which are not just on the true to false spectrum. Some help us all to live despite "reality."

Pessoa's devotion to a painful sense of and an arrogant pride in being nothing yet always being astonished by human sensations and ideas is illustrated in many of his poems. The following poem, for example, makes the ironical point that to see oneself as worthless is a value. Paradox is something of profound ontological significance to this plural poet.

> Well, now that I am alone and can see
> With the heart's power to discern
> How much I am not, how much I cannot be
> How much, if I became it, I should be in vain
>
> Now, I will confess, I want to feel
> Once and for all I am no one,
> And to proudly resign from myself
> For not having acted well
>
> I failed in everything, though without trying;
> I have been nothing, dared nothing, done nothing,
> Nor did I pluck from the nettles of my days
> The flower of seeming-happiness
>
> But there always remains, because whoever is poor
> Is rich in something, if one looks properly,
> The great indifference which is left me
> I note this to remember it without fail{PM: End indent}

It is somewhat important to record in an article of this kind that Pessoa saw himself as a leader of an intellectual cult in

Portuguese life, which was called sensationism. He crudely put it, "There is nothing but sensation." To some extent, though not explicitly, this is akin to David Hume's (1711–1776) description of human experience as analogous to a series of essentially disconnected kaleidoscopic images. These views are perhaps best presented in his notes on sensationism, which show the influence of Spinoza:

> "Spinoza said that philosophical systems are right in what they affirm and wrong in what they deny. This, the greatest of all pantheistic affirmations, is what sensationism can repeat in relation to aesthetic things. Though supreme perfection (which is unattainable) is only one (. . .) relative perfection is several. Homer is as perfect in his way as Herrick in his, although the Homeric way is a far superior one. The sensationist joyfully admits both Homer and Herrick to the great brotherhood of Art."

There are three central tenets of sensationism. The first is that art is supremely construction and that the greatest art is the one that is able to visualize and create organized wholes, of which the component parts fit vitally into their places; the great principle that Aristotle enunciated when he said that a poem was an "animal." The second is that since all art is composed of parts, each of those parts must be perfect in itself. As the first tenet is the classical principle of unity and structural perfection, this second one is the romantic principle of "fine passages." That would make those sufficient for what they contain of truth and exclude the error that makes of all this, without attending to the higher classical principle, that the whole is greater than the part. The third tenet of sensationism, qua aesthetics, is that every little fragment which builds up the part of the whole should be perfect in itself. This is the principle that is the symbolist artists insist on to the point of exaggeration. Since they are temperamentally incapable of creating either great organized wholes or even (like the Romantics) large eloquent stretches, they put their activity into the eggshell (nutshell) of producing beautiful individual lines or very short, perfect lyrics. That is beautiful indeed, when it is beautiful, but it is dangerous to fall under the impression that is anything but the lowest part of art.

These are the tenets of sensationism qua artistic philosophy. That is to say, these are the tenets it upholds, although it accepts all systems and schools of art, extracting from each that beauty and originality which is peculiar to it.

Sensationism stands for the aesthetic attitude in all its pagan splendor. It does not stand for any of those other foolish things, such as the aestheticism of Oscar Wilde or the art for art's sake of other misguided people with a plebeian outlook on life. It can see the loveliness of morals just as it can understand the beauty of the lack of them. No religion is right for it, nor any religion wrong.

A man may traverse all the religious systems of the world in one day with perfect sincerity and tragic soul experiences. He must be an aristocrat – in the true sense of the word – to be able to do it. I once stated that a cultured and intelligent man has the duty to be into all things, and an ultramontane catholic at that precise hour after sunset when the shadows have not yet completed their slow coil round the clear presence of things. Some people thought that this was a joke. But I was only translating into rapid prose (this was written in a newspaper) a common personal experience. Having accustomed myself to having no beliefs and no opinions, lest my aesthetic feeling should be weakened, I soon grew to have no personality at all except an expressive one. I grew to be a mere apt machine for the expression of moods that became so intense that they grew into personalities and made my very soul the mere shell of their casual appearance, even as theosophists say that the malice of nature-spirits sometimes makes them occupy the discarded astral corpses of men and frolic under cover of their shadowy semblances (substances).

This does not mean that every sensationist should have no political opinions; it means that, as an artist, he is bound to have none and all. That excuse of Martial's, which has aroused the ire of many people alien to the essence of art – "Lasciva est nobis pagina, vita proba" – that though his art was impure, his life was not (reproduced later by Herrick, who wrote of himself, "His muse was jocund, but his life was chaste"), is the exact duty of the artist towards himself.

Sincerity is the one great artistic crime. Insincerity is the second greatest. The great artist should never have a really fundamental and sincere opinion about life. But that should give him the capacity to feel sincere, nay, to be absolutely sincere about anything for a certain length of time – that length of time, say, which is necessary for a poem to be conceived and written. It is perhaps necessary to state that it is necessary to be an artist before this can be attempted. It is of no use to try to be an aristocrat when you are a born middle-class man or plebeian.

Pessoa also shows a perspicacious attitude toward scientific nomenclature, one which pervades psychiatric taxonomy: "When a classification is for a certain purpose, either practical or scientific, it will necessarily be arbitrary (philosophically) and contingent upon the end for which it is made." (Note: Pessoa is addressing scientific nomenclature in general, and not specifically psychiatric taxonomy). The botanist and the gardener both need a different classification for plants». The question of the existence of a correct classification to be discovered, perhaps as Monads or fundamental particles of physics, remains a philosophical issue. For the practice of psychiatry in any century near ours, there is necessarily something political about what is socially accepted. It is that which legitimizes all the acts practiced on labeled persons.

There is "political conflict" about what is sacred and what is mad, especially when faced with borderline life, artistic creation, and love. The social collective is forced to define itself in the light of discordances it must confront in the fundamentals of its own culture. It responds by domesticating, and that process begins by assigning a name, a code, and a number. This is a strategy of the intellectually sophisticated. Another Portuguese writer, Teixeira de Pascoes (1877–1952), asserts that to give vacuous names to things full of meaning (. . .) Delusions! Hallucinations! But rationality and hallucinations are derived from the same fountain as that from which springs the verses of Homer and the stones of the pyramids. Everything has the same vital energy, the same vague vibration, as giving a name which says nothing.

Certainly, the presumption of most schools of psychiatry is not only the necessity but the legitimacy of psychiatric classifications, and that is presumed to be for scientific and medical reasons rather than political ones. So, on this we can give Pessoa's further words: "All scientific classification is useful, clear, and always false."

We have struggled to illustrate the outlook of the genius creator Fernando Pessoa and its relevance to psychiatry. Here we have selected from Pessoan poetry and a few commentaries in the inimitable ironic and somewhat paradoxical way that the poet wove his web around psychiatry. The appearance of consciousness, or, if you prefer, the ability of matter to subsequently perceive itself aesthetically remains the great "incognito." We would like to end by quoting Fernando Pessoa on this fact of a thoughtless universe developing thinking.

After all there is no difference
If the flowers bloom without wanting to
Without wanting to we think
What in it is blooming
In us is to be conscious

In homage to Fernando Pessoa, we can also contemplate the poem "Autopsychography, where the author tells us that he thinks a poet is no longer a maker (poiesis) but a faker:

Autopsychography

The poet is a faker. He
Fakes it so completely,
He even fakes he's suffering
The pain he's really feeling

And they who read his writing
Fully feel while reading
Not that pain of his that's double,
But theirs, completely fictional

So on its tracks goes round and round,
To entertain the reason,
That wound-up little train
We call the heart of man

Translations of the poems are from E. Honig and S M Brown. They can capture only the meaning and, as closely as possible, the poetry.

4. Psychiatrizing Society and Panopticism

No one should overlook the dangers of society psychiatrizing itself any more than one should miss the point that societies first defined madness and gave it to psychiatry. We present some issues of the psychologized society and look at them in the light of panopticism.

We analyze the possible articulation between psychiatrized society, power, and the symbols linked to them. We look on power positively, in the manner of Michel Foucault, and analyze its importance to the community, in the light of Bentham's "Panoptic."

All the philosophical, ethical, and biological arguments of the liberal discourse separating the world of "rationality-freedom-productivity" from the world of "madness-irresponsibility-leisure" had an economic base. Madness was a problem for the capitalist society of the eighteenth century because the unproductivity of the madman offended the new "religion of work," which was considered "the" means to achieve humanity and freedom. But, as we know, the revolutions in the world can result in laments like "Freedom, what crimes are committed in your name."

Indeed, mental hospitals expanded greatly after the Liberal Revolution. Some people who defend and maintain mental hospitals ignore or pretend to ignore the fact that they, and not the "patients," are the real clients of those institutions. As Erving Goffman (1961) puts it, mental hospitals do not exist just because the directors, psychiatrists, and nurses need a job or some employment. They exist because there is a specific market for them: if all the mental hospitals of some country were emptied and closed, sooner or later, the patients' families, the police, and tribunals would ask for them to open again, because those real clients of mental hospitals need this kind of institution to fulfil their needs. This means that the "functions" of mental hospitals are not exactly to treat some "diseases," but to solve some (social) "problems."

One of the ironic triumphs of the age of reason was to replace the leper houses with places of confinement for a new category of outsider. The true intention was not medical but judicial, "correction through confinement."

We do agree that some institutions are tools of the Modern State, developed to solve "problems." Society needs courts and a concept of "justice" in order to defend ownership of property, but inevitably to pronounce on "responsibility," about which we know nothing. We are, nevertheless, doomed to play games like those of "justice."

Psychiatry, like justice, needs concepts. Psychiatry is based on concepts of proper ideas and behavior and, at a basic level, a series of value judgments about beliefs and comportment. They are ethical or, even more accurately, ethics disguised as science.

In psychiatry, the concepts are not facts but value judgments, which is another version of the "good and bad" moral dichotomy transformed into the "normal and pathological" medical one. Perhaps to some extent, as there are good paintings, there are good ideas in psychiatry, healthy thoughts, but less often quite correct ones.

In the Archeology of Knowledge, Michel Foucault describes the means of making scientific objects, methods, and theories. We agree with him that many recognizable objects are not natural ones but are made by man (us), through words. In this sense, the thought is prisoner of the discourse, in which words do not represent things tout court (the name is not the named thing). The objects are brought up from the relationship net between phenomena (the problem) in order to act upon it: a knowledge has/is power. There are not facts per se but socially constructed objects. Not very differently, in this respect, Henry Bergson, the spiritualist and vitalist philosopher, believed that, in the end, science is no more than fiction constructed to serve some social "conveniences."

Ludwig Wittgenstein (1976) suggested that grammar may be a significantly more arbitrary sociohistorical product than cooking, but one upon which logic is based. This seems consistent with an overall socially based ideology that is defended against thoroughgoing nominalism or relativism by Wittgenstein's point that the importance of ideas comes from more than language; indeed, it comes from the human need to believe what is congenial. What has been indoctrinated and, of course, what is realistic about cooking and living in general, for us, are successful technological or pragmatic ways of doing things.

Conceptualization may be influenced by the environment almost as much as enunciation and may be almost as difficult to escape. "Right" and "wrong," "good" and "bad," "just" and "unjust," "saint" and "sinner," "tables" and "chairs," and later, if learning psychiatry, "schizophrenia," are all words one must struggle to use, or to understand as others do. Where "desks" become "tables," "stools" become "chairs," and "streams" "rivers," are as contingent on human beings as, for instance, the border between Portugal and Spain (especially in Galicia, where the Galaico-Portuguese language is spoken) or England and Scotland. Now the demarcations are essentially agreed on, even if those living in Berwick on Tweed might prefer to be in Berwickshire. From the viewpoint of Wittgenstein (1976), it is, nevertheless, right to point out that: "It is possible to call us nominalists if we are not conscious that a boundary drawn by a definition is drawn only for the sake of the importance of this boundary. And the propositions which explain the importance are not propositions about language." We take that to mean that language has to function for us and serve our purposes. It could not do so if delineations were totally independent of what serves our purposes or did not therefore take into account realities and possibilities in the world. Wittgenstein saw that constraint as being less on grammar than on vocabulary.

Drawing a border between "normality" and "madness" is a historical procedure based on ideo-moral and ethical-political judgments.

Power is invested in all scientific practices in several ways through the judicial-institutional organization and its ideological and material dispositions. In the case of psychiatry, this relationship of dependence is too obvious and allows us to understand why psychopathological practices have not developed, until now, a critical and internal consciousness, which could show its instrumentality by power, and its role as a normalizing process. The psychiatric management of "madness" serves the political strategies to normalize people, and hence madness cannot be looked at as a possible way of being human, that is, as an "alternative psychology" (Jenner et al., 1993).

Thomas Szasz (1971) argues that the involuntary patient in psychiatry makes its practice an extension of the law and that its drugs are chemical straitjackets. However, psychiatry does not operate only inside the walls of asylums. It extends its power to other and vaster realities. There is a recognizable psychopathologization of human behavior, and too many things are codified in psychopathological terms or diagnoses. This has the effect of applying psychopathological language and diagnoses to literature, the arts, historical events, sociocultural phenomena, political facts, and politicians or others. We believe this effect is the domestication of "things full of meaning" (Teixeira de Pascoes), such as political contestation, marginalities, artistic creation, experience of the sacred, falling in love, madness, and all the historical phenomena and human experiences that do not perform properly in the game of the Modern State and its power interests but cannot be checked by other "names," diagnostic numbers, and classifications given to them. To paraphrase Foucault (1961), we must always remember that the person who confesses himself supplies the "raw data," but it is the father confessor who gives the "correct meaning."

The implication that domestication of the individual may be inevitable is plain to see. In that case, resisting for as long as possible is the only possible strategy. For instance, psychoanalysis is reducing people to sets of determined psychodynamic laws and thereby denying their freedom and responsibility. In addition, even now it pretends that a massive amount of training improves therapeutic skills. The current psychotherapeutic epidemic shows hegemony (the rule by the dominant class that controls the thoughts of others).

A leading Portuguese psychoanalyst wrote, "The mission of mental health professionals is to impose rationality on the world" (Carlos A. A. Dias). Similarly, as the motto of the X World Congress of Psychiatry (Madrid, August 1996) implied, "One Language, One World." But, we ask, which language and which world? Of course, we are told of the virtues of an international and shared language for research purposes; journal readers will at last be able to recognize the operational definitions used. But Szasz (1977) had already dealt with all that quite well in The Manufacture of Madness, which we would render as suggesting that if we read of a group of Benedictine Monks preparing the Malleus Mallificarum with the same arguments, we might accept the view that a Babel of languages can be better than dogma. The Malleus Mallificarum served as a powerful definition of witches because it had a powerful backing. The PSE, DSM-IV (American Psychiatric Association), DC-10 (World Health Organization), and Feignher et al. systems are similar concepts and came in one way or another from Kraepelin via Schneider, even though Schneider warned us against using first rank symptoms as diagnostic signs. He said they were an arbitrary typology he used!

We realize that looking for mental diseases before Kraepelin, Jaspers, Bleuler, Freud, Schneider, DMS IV, DC 10, Feignher, etc., constituted them would be as useless as looking for transgressions of the Napoleonic Code before it was instituted (1980). In our view, it would be very surprising to find, outside the rationalization of power of the Modern State, the most specific consequences of the predominant sociocultural conditions in the last two centuries in the so-called Western World: the systematic eradication of the unforeseeable, the spontaneous, and the irrational. Thus, mental diseases are close relatives of transgressions of criminal and civil law from the nineteenth century onward.

It is interesting to recall the famous faetor judaicus, a particular kind of smell that came from classical antiquity to the seventeenth century, and which some educated people and inquisitors noticed in Jews. For Father Cristovão de Santo Tirso, the generation of Jews was fetid, as were their errors. The case became more complicated when Vicente da Costa, in 1668, in

Lisbon, asserted that baptized Jews lost the smell of their bodies but that they regained their particular smell as soon as they apostatized from the Christian religion. He explained, "Some serious doctors say that this fetidness was natural in all those who participated in Our Lord's death" (Sampaio Bruno, 1983). Therefore, there is reason to remark that, at that time, genetic theories about such a smell already prevailed, even though the genetic imperfections could be manipulated by religious means. As we know, some years ago, lots of psychiatrists allowed themselves to be seduced by the usefulness of a particular smell as a diagnostic criterion for schizophrenia.

Recently, the leading Portuguese family therapist, Daniel Sampaio, commented on a TV talk show that: "There are mothers and fathers by chance that are the result of unplanned affective relationships." If they had been planned, we think they would not be affective relations but rational ones. This is really another way to impose rationality on the world.

There are now technical, psychological, and apparently soft neologisms, such as "deviation" and "deviant behavior" in place of the words "disease" and "illness." We can certainly ask to whom and to what criteria they are related. Indeed, "disease" and "deviations" are, in this context, words to qualify the variability and the diversity of human behavior. They have the same social meaning and function for the domesticating process. Certainly, those words are tools for purposes ... What we have at hand does give some authority to doctors and psychologists. It allows them to domesticate unpredictable and socially threatening behavior.

In a society dominated by what we call the Normalization Utopian Project, in which genetics is particularly prominent in scientific explanations and a particular importance is attached to understanding that any tendency to consider a human being as a product of genetic determinism risks denying the fact that the person also has an enormous genetically conferred plasticity and variability which confers a great richness and diversity which is so particularly sui generis.

Symbols are compact representations of philosophies and ideologies that play a socially reproductive role. Different areas of human activity and social praxis are crammed with symbols. For this reason, we can analyze the symbols and social organization of the Modern Post-Industrial Revolution State. The symbolic is influenced by daily life and the Zeitgeist of the social-historical context.

The era of "orthopaedic obsession" (upright position), started, in general, by the occidental rationalist societies, persists, but are the actual communities not far from the clarity and scientific optimism that thought it had the power to correct and prevent deformations of body and soul?

The era in which the child must listen and be seen but not heard is illustrated by the rebel tree that seems to refuse to grow vertically.

In the model of calligraphy of the Model College of Navarra, all the gestures, movements, and positions obey fixed predetermined rules, which discipline, normalize, and adapt bodies and minds for socioeconomic purposes.

The democratizing society of producers/consumers (A. Toffler: Prosumers) is competitive, mathematical, and disciplined. This society can be represented symbolically by the Panopticism of Jeremy Bentham.

We live in a disciplining community with micropowers and microknowledges that normalize functions. The symbolic representation of this type of society can be the Bentham Panoptic. The panoptic is a building in the shape of a ring, which has a central yard with a tower in the middle. The ring is divided into small cells, fully illuminated by day and by night. In the central tower there is a strategic position, from which a vigilant person can observe all that can happen. Each cell is occupied by a worker working, a prisoner serving a term, a fool producing delusions, or a child learning social rules; respectively, a factory, a jail, an asylum, or a school. The Benthamite architectural model can also be used for zoos, museums, state buildings, military quarters, nurseries, shopping centers, towns, cities, etc.

The eye can be the symbol of the panoptic tower. The functional success is based on the principals of circularity and clearness. Those principles allow the vigilant to see all the gestures of the people exposed without being seen themselves. (Isn't that like psychoanalysis?)

Societies organized as Modern States follow the disciplinary panoptic model completely, connecting the panoptic power, the panoptic community, and the panoptic symbol. The panoptic look avoids the social emancipation of human beings under the eye of the "Episcopal" successors. (Etymology: Latin Episcopu is from epi, meaning above, and from skope, meaning to see or observe, in the sense of controlling; Greek Episkopos means ancient Greek magistrate who inspected a certain circumscribed territory called a diocese.) The actual Episcopal successors have the sophisticated panoptic resources of the informatics, genetic, and molecular era.

M. Foucault says that the power is a magnetic and never-ending infiltration of the social field. This means the panoptic systems or panopticism (omniseeing, omnicontrol, and omnipower).

The panoptic by itself imprints its management onto bodies, minds, time, space, relationships in the community. In the panoptic model of social organization, vigilance is automatic; it is experienced with or without somebody in the central tower. The look produces the effects of the power. The vigilant does not have a real existence but a symbolic one. The tower of vigilance symbolizes the vigilant himself. By this symbolization, the vigilant gets a real existence in the consciousness of the one who is watched. That is the way to self-vigilance (or internal locus of control). In a panoptic community, there is no need for walls. As Foucault (1979) puts it, "a real submission is born automatically from a fictitious relationship," or, as Roland Barthes (1979) said, "It is not only to tolerate power but also to sympathize with it."

Michel Foucault says the panoptic must be understood not as a building but as a diagram of the "power mechanism in its ideal form." Panopticism is enriched by new technologies of the era of informatics, by case registers, by profiles, by epidemiological psychiatric studies, by spy satellites, etc. Panopticism puts rationality in an arousal state to dismiss the temptation, deviance, and differences always present.

The orthopaedic obsession of panopticism is supported by a relevant contribution of the young human sciences (psychology, psychoanalysis, psychiatry, pedagogy, testology, etc.).

In a panoptic community, knowledge and power are not dissociated. The exam is the bridge which links the panoptic to scientific knowledge. Psychiatric, psychological, pedagogic, professional, military, and scientific examinations and their rituals, methods, actors, and roles produce systems of social classification and hierarchies. Social organization of asylums as means of examination preceded the emergence of the first books of psychiatry. The examination makes the individual an analyzable and isolated object. Scientific method makes a case of each individual and desubjectivizes it through a "degradation ceremony" in its underlying classificatory framework.

Examination and experimentation are not everyday situations but artificial ones. For example, Harlow, between 1954 and 1957, searched for "nature love" through experiences in laboratories.

Here, as in other situations, perhaps Wittgenstein is right: object and method are too far one from another.

Natural philosophy, or epistemology, is also part of the panoptic eye that controls and sometimes blames science and also philosophy.

The panoptic is the symbol of the utopia of a society and of a power. This utopia is actually achieved in our society. It is organized in the form of a Modern State.

Panopticism can be illustrated by Salvador Dali's painting "Giraffe in Flames." This picture presents the orthopaedic obsession shown by the brace of power (the image of the thin body that is standing up but with the help of a machine or external support). As we know, Salvador Dali was classified as a surrealist; it is easier to classify him than to contemplate his mystery.

In panopticism, the "Pathology of the Spirit" is a means to foresee the psychological truth about human beings and to objectify it.

Will the towns of the future be vertical, panoptical, clear, and circular ones?

Panopticism and its consequent application of rational thought to social organization produces the social marginalization and exclusion of those who do not have the social and cultural norms of the mainstream or do not have personal or social success (Alain Touraine, 1992).

The experiences of "schizophrenia," being enamored of something or somebody, and feeling inspired by the sacred can be viewed as "nascent states," in the sense of Francesco Alberoni (1983). Society has utopian plans, in the sense of Baczko (1985), in relation to the "nascent states." Hence the attempt is made to domesticate, neutralize, and institutionalize them in church and in asylums. Clearly, the "nascent states" disrupt any power based on rationality,

Fernando Pessoa (1976) conceptualized mankind quite differently than Aristotle. Pessoa wrote: "Emotion and not reason controls man as it does animals . . . Science and reason preside as a constitutional monarch, who reigns but does not govern. Human action is irrational, contradictory, and absurd . . . reason illuminates a way; it does not determine it."

We certainly agree that all "nascent states" have a great potential for disorder and chaos that is incompatible with the maintenance and stability of the Modern State. Certainly, we also realize that all these "nascent states" release conflict and instability, particularisms and unforeseeable circumstances. They release all that the central power wishes to regulate.

If the role of the Modern State is to impose a rational structure on communities in which the traditional lack of structure is always latent, then there is a need for legitimacy, which was previously derived from a universal and state religion. With power going into the hands of the laity, the place of this religion was taken up by what is understood as science, and in this sense scientific knowledge began to legitimize the requirements of power and thereby dominate and regulate the so-called conflicts.

As psychiatrists, it is particularly important to understand which conflicts we are given the power to dominate and regulate: small rational conflicts and those which are determined by "nascent states." This is the panoptic object of psychiatric biochemistry, genetics, and biostatistics.

The dominance of the genetics and biochemistry of human beings accused of being ill can only lead to a panoptic society of look-alikes: inhuman, cold, without conflicts, without emotions, without greatness. To paraphrase Dodds (1951), "a place where everything is so terribly rational."

We think that the mandate that society has historically given to, or that medicine has taken for, psychiatry, etymological medicine of the mind in relation to the mental health services, stretches much more questionably beyond the limits of the so-called psychoses. The wisdom of Fernando Pessoa is correct, and the panoptic function of psychiatry can be foreseen in the way Pessoa (1976) puts it:

> "In reality the unique critics of art and literature ought to be the psychiatrists: although they are as ignorant about these issues and as remote from them and from what they call science as other people, nevertheless, when faced with mental disease they have the competence that our judgment says they have. No body of human knowledge can be built on any other bases" (written in 1915).

In a sense, Pessoa made it clear that he saw psychopathology as a socially legitimated ideology, which meant nothing ontologically.

Glossary

Epidemiology: the study of trends, e.g., in data
Nascent: in the act of coming into existence; beginning to form or grow
Nominalism: the view that regards universals and abstract concepts as mere names without any corresponding realities
Ontology: the study of what is so, irrespective of us
Relativism: the view that there are no universal standards of good and bad, right and wrong
Sui generis: peculiar to its own kind
Zeitgeist: the thought or feeling peculiar to a generation or period

Bibliography

Alberoni, F. 1983. Enamoramento e Amor. Translated by A. Puga. Amadora: Bertrand.

Baczko. 1985. "Utopia." In Enciclopédia Einaudi 5:333–96.

Barthes, R. 1977. Fragments d' un discour amoreux. Paris: Editions du Seuil.

Bentham, J. 1979. Le Panoptic. In L'Oeil du Pouvoir, edited by M. Foucault. Paris: Editions Pierre Belfond.

Cardoso, Herménio. 1952. Tese para provas de doutoramento em Medicina. Edição do Autor: Coimbra.

Dodds, E. R. 1951. The Greeks and the Irrational. Harmondsworth: Pelican Books.

Pessoa, Fernando. 1976. O Rosto e as Máscaras: Textos Escolhidos em Verso e Prosa (Org. David Mourão Ferreira). Lisboa: Círculo dos Leitores.

Foucault, M. 1972. Histoire de la Folie à l' Âge Classique. Paris: Gallimard.

———. 1975. Surveiller et Punir. Paris: Gallimard.

———. 1976. La Volonté de Savoir (Histoire de la Sexualité I). Paris: Gallimard.

———. 1979. L'Oeil du Pouvoir. Paris: Editions Pierre Belfond.

Goffman, E. 1961. Asylums: Essays on the Social Situation of Mental Patients and Other Inmates. New York: Anchor.

Jenner, F. A., A. Monteiro, J. A. Zagalo-Cardoso, and Cunha-Oliveira. 1993. Schizophrenia: A Disease or Some Ways of Being Human? Sheffield: Sheffield Academic Press.

Sampaio-Bruno. 1983. O Encoberto. Porto: Lello e Irmão.

Szasz, Th. 1971. The Manufacture of Madness: A Comparative Studyof the Inquisition and the Mental Health Movement. New York: Harper and Row.

———. 1977. Schizophrenia: The Sacred Symbol of Psychiatry. New York: Basic Books Publisher.

Touraine, A. 1992. Critique de la Modernité. Paris: Librairie Arthéme Fayard.

Wittgenstein, L. (1976). Philosophical Investigations. Translated by G. E. M. Oxford: Basic Blackwell.

Zagalo-Cardoso, J. A. 1993. "Fernando Pessoa (1888–1935): The Portuguese Poet and Philosopher." Asylum 7(1):10–12.

*If you loved this book, would you please
submit a review at Amazon.com?*

www.ingramcontent.com/pod-product-compliance
Lightning Source LLC
Chambersburg PA
CBHW021042180526
45163CB00005B/2249